So Young, So Sad, So Listen

So Young, So Sad, So Listen

By
Philip Graham and Carol Hughes

Drawings by
Christine Roche

Foreword by
Philip Pullman

Oh WHERE
Oh WHERE
has my little
spark gone...

GASKELL

Gaskell is an imprint of The Royal College of Psychiatrists,
17 Belgrave Square, London SW1X 8PG
http://www.rcpsych.ac.uk

British Library Cataloguing-in-Publication Data
A catalogue record for this book is available from the British Library.
ISBN 1-904671-23-3

Distributed in North America by Balogh International Inc.

Acknowledgement

We thank the West London Health Promotion Agency for their
support in producing the first edition of this book. Thanks also
to Raphael Kelvin for updating some sections of the text in 2008.

Printed in Great Britain by Cromwell Press Limited, Trowbridge, Wiltshire

Contents

Foreword

Depression: it hardly sounds like an illness, does it? It sounds like a mood. It sounds like something you could snap out of, with a bit of will power; like something you'd have to be feeble to give in to.

Our ancestors called it melancolia, or melancholy – but even melancholy sounds mild. It sounds like the sort of pleasing gentle sadness we might feel in autumn as we see the leaves turn brown and fall from the trees.

None of these names does it justice. There's nothing mild or gentle about what we call depression. In fact, at its worst it's a savage and merciless disease. Those of us who have felt its power dread it and shun it, and know the way it can ravage and torment the mind, and pursue us unrelentingly while shutting off every avenue of escape, until there seems to be only one way out of the dark labyrinth we're trapped in: and that way is suicide.

It's a horrible thing to suffer from. It's bad enough for adults, although people who've had brushes with it can develop ways of coping when they sense it lurking nearby. Keeping busy helps, and taking exercise, and not spending too much time on our own, or in gloomy surroundings.

But it can catch children in its grip, too. Young people are just as susceptible, and it's harder for them, because they have nothing to compare it with; and sometimes it strikes when they are going through adolescence, that most confusing and stressful period, when their bodies are changing rapidly, when they are beset by all kinds of social and personal embarrassments, when sexual feelings are increasingly urgent, when every relationship is under strain. Sometimes the starting point of a bout of depression might be family problems that seem impossible to deal with – divorce, bereavement, or an abusive adult; but sometimes it strikes out of the blue, with hardly any apparent reason. Whatever the cause and wherever it comes from, if depression strikes when you're young, it strikes very hard indeed.

Why it affects some and not others is still a mystery. The important thing to remember is that there are ways to deal with it. One of the most deadly tricks of this cunning and malevolent disease is to persuade us that the hopeless despair we're suffering is our fault: that we are somehow to blame for the state we're in, that we don't deserve to live and be happy.

This is where the informed help of other people can be so important. This book is full of helpful information not only for the young sufferer, but for their friends, and for parents and teachers and other adults who deal with children. I'm glad that such a source of good advice and information exists, and I hope it will lighten many burdens.

Philip Pullman

Introduction

This book is about depression in children and teenagers during their school years, from 5 to 16. It is written for parents and teachers. We also hope that social workers, health visitors and family doctors will find it useful. Perhaps some teenagers themselves might find it interesting.

Do children and young teenagers really get depressed? Here are four accounts of depression about four different children, described by a mother, a teacher, a psychiatrist and a 14-year-old girl herself. (The names and some details have been changed.) These are followed by descriptions of childhood depression remembered in adulthood.

The mother

Ben's mother, an art teacher, describes the change that came over him after a short viral illness.

> 'He changed somehow. The change was so gradual that it was hard to pinpoint at first. We thought he was still recovering from the virus and took him to the doctor. But, slowly, we became aware that things were getting worse. He seemed to have lost his sparkle – he used to be such a lively, interested and interesting 10-year-old, with a passion for Arsenal! Then even football lost its charm for him. We felt he was just going through the motions of everyday life. He would agree to most things, but do them without enjoyment. He quickly became tearful over minor incidents. He stayed indoors more and more and we realised that he spoke less frequently about his friends or their joint activities. Unless we pushed him into doing some activity, he would just do nothing. It was such an upsetting difference from the energetic, sometimes exhausting, lively child that we had known.'

The teacher

Angela is an intelligent 8-year-old girl whom her teacher thought of as a 'real pain' in the classroom. In a reasonably well-behaved class of 32 children, she was very much the odd one out. Some of the other children, especially the boys, were amused by the way she made peculiar noises when the class was supposed to be quiet, but most of the others, like her teacher, were irritated by the way she drew attention to herself. Angela, when not being disruptive, would sit looking out of the window, apparently in a world of her own. In the playground she would mix with a group of young children, sometimes pushing them around and hurting them, so that teachers had to intervene. Although Angela's mother had previously denied any problem with her at home, on the next occasion the teacher saw her she decided to press more firmly on the subject. Eventually, tears came to Angela's mother's eyes and she explained how her husband had been made redundant, was drinking heavily, and was himself depressed. Money was very, very tight. Angela was his favourite of the four children, but now he had little time for her and would push her away when she tried to sit on his knee. The mother herself was worried about Angela, who was not at all naughty at home, but miserable and listless, not wanting to play with her friends, and sometimes saying she wished she were dead.

At the teacher's suggestion, through her general practitioner, Angela was referred to the local child and family psychiatric clinic. The family members were seen together on three occasions and Angela's father was able to talk about his sense of failure. The family problems remained considerable, but Angela now seemed to understand the situation, was more settled and less miserable, wanted to play with her friends and was much less trouble in class.

The psychiatrist

Harry was a 13-year-old boy who had started to get into trouble – quite serious trouble – when he transferred from primary to secondary school. He had been one of the leading lights in his final year at primary school, but on beginning secondary school he had started to become irritable and difficult. By the following year he had got involved with a couple of boys who had been trouble-makers since early childhood and were a real nuisance in the neighbourhood, breaking into cars, stealing from shops and truanting from school. Eventually, he was charged with breaking and entering property and a psychiatric report was requested. The psychiatrist found him to be a seriously depressed boy. He had been transferred away from the good friends he had made at primary school to a different secondary school, which was some way from his home. He found the work more difficult and was discouraged by failure. In addition, at home his mother had developed depression herself and was unable to prepare meals or do the housework. His father had left home some years previously. Under a tough exterior, Harry admitted he had long periods of misery when he thought about his father and wondered how he could get in touch with him. He wanted to be helpful at home, but did not know how. He felt angry with the world, but also with himself. Practical help from a probation officer to get his mother to the doctor for her depression and back to the job she had given up, extra help for Harry at school and contact with a sports centre made a real difference to Harry's behaviour.

The teenager

Anna was a 14-year-old girl who described her depression very movingly.

'I felt as though no one could like me. I began to wonder just what was the point of anything. At first I lost interest in everything. I felt tired all the time and didn't sleep properly. I would wake up before the rest of the family and lie there feeling grotty and forgotten by the whole world. It felt as if everything was darkness and full of nothing, stretching out to the horizon and filling every corner.'

Adults looking back

When adults look back on their childhood, they sometimes describe clear episodes of depression. Sir Peter Hall, the theatre director and founder of the Royal Shakespeare Company, describes in his auto-biography *Making an Exhibition of Myself* (published by Sinclair-Stevenson, London, 1994) how he has, from time to time in his life, become suicidally depressed. On the first occasion he was 8 years old. His family had moved from a small village to what seemed to him the big city of Cambridge. He writes:

'I have felt suicidal several times ... this was the first time it struck and perhaps because I had fewer inner resources and less to distract me than when I was grown up, it was perhaps the worst time of all. I was very near the brink... I was sent to the elementary school just around the corner... I, an only child of eight and a loner from the wilds of Suffolk, was mocked by brawling boys and giggling girls. Perhaps it was because of my Suffolk burr. I remember how the children listened to me and then burst out laughing... My depression was acute and today would be considered very dangerous. I survived, as I was always to survive, by frantic activity. I gradually came back from the brink.'

The poet Sylvia Plath took her own life in 1962, when she was in her early 30s. It is clear that she had had depressive episodes in which she at least contemplated and maybe attempted suicide since she was about 10 years old. One of her last poems, Lady Lazarus, begins 'I have done it again./One year in every ten/I manage it –' (*Ariel*, published by Faber & Faber, London, 1965).

We should make it clear there is no evidence that people who are very creative are more likely to suffer depression than others. But they have their share of depression, and when they are affected they are, of course, particularly good at describing what it feels like.

Attitudes to children with depression

So children and teenagers do get depressed. Parents and teachers, when they hear about a child who might be depressed, think to themselves: 'They're just too young for that to happen'. But, as you can see from these examples, they are certainly not too young. It is not helpful to deny that the young can get depressed. That attitude usually means that we close our eyes and pretend that it is not happening, even when it clearly is.

Another attitude can be summed up as: 'Oh, how awful, poor thing. It upsets me terribly just to think about it. How dreadful for the parents. How guilty they must be'. That is not very helpful either. Depressed children and teenagers do need sympathy, but this is not enough. Furthermore, although troubles at home are sometimes the cause of depression, there are many other causes, some in school (as Peter Hall's example shows) and some in the child's or teenager's personality.

Depression in childhood and early adolescence is a fact of life we have to face. It is sad, but there is often a good deal that can be done to help, providing we recognise that the problem exists, and providing that we do not jump to conclusions too quickly about what is causing it.

In this book we have tried to give useful information about depression in young people. It is, in fact, one of the most common, serious problems in today's school-age population. We have tried to describe how depression can be recognised by parents, teachers and young people themselves. We then explain what can be done to help.

1 What is depression?

Everyone recognises that children and young people of any age can be sad and miserable. Disappointments and frustrations, some big and some small, are common in all young lives. Furthermore, we all recognise that when sadness and misery are prolonged, children and teenagers can be really distressed. However, it is only relatively recently, in the past 20 years or so, that it has become clear that a significant number of children and teenagers (see chapter 3) have such serious disturbances of mood that it is quite appropriate to think of them as having depressive disorders.

There is no clear dividing line between children and young people who are very sad and miserable and those who are clinically depressed. Obviously, a child whose pet dog has just died and who is really upset for several days is not clinically depressed, whereas another who has been mute, refusing to eat or speak, and is thinking of suicide is suffering from an illness, not just an ordinary mood change. But in many cases, the distinction is nowhere near as easy as this to make.

Although serious depression in a child or teenager may indeed sometimes be best seen as a disorder or even an illness, this is by no means the only way to look at it. Depression in a young person may be a sign that something is very wrong in the family or the school or in the neighbourhood. Social, educational, and family perspectives on depression are sometimes more appropriate than seeing it as a disorder or a medical problem. We hope this will become clear after we have described the ways depression in the young can occur.

Every 10 or 15 years the World Health Organization publishes guidelines for doctors, psychologists and nurses on the ways in which it is internationally agreed that diagnoses should be made. In the latest version, published in 1992, there is guidance that depression in childhood and adolescence should be diagnosed in the same way as in adults. Obviously, the sorts of stresses experienced by children and young people are different from those in adults, but in our experience the World Health Organization is right. Although the stresses are different, the ways in which children, young people and adults show depression are really very similar – not identical, but in many ways the same.

2 Signs of depression

Sad, unhappy mood

The child or young person with depression will show sadness and misery for weeks at a time, with little variation from day to day, although the mood might change during the day. Even though circumstances may alter, the sad mood may persist.

Recognising a persistently unhappy mood may not be easy. The boy or girl may experience a mood change, but not want to admit it. As we describe below, children and young people who are depressed may have other problems, such as difficult, disobedient or even aggressive behaviour. It is particularly hard for parents and teachers to recognise persistently sad mood in a child who is being disruptive. By no means all disruptive, difficult children are depressed, but a sizeable number of them are.

Depression is sometimes also accompanied by anxiety, and this may show itself with aches and pains, especially stomach-aches and headaches which are difficult to diagnose. If a parent is worried that there may be something physically wrong with the child, the accompanying depressed mood may well be overlooked.

Lack of pleasure in ordinary, everyday activities

Most children and teenagers will say that they get bored sometimes. They usually mean they get bored when there is nothing to do, when, for example, their friends are away or do not call for them, or when the computer has crashed or when the weather is bad and they cannot play football. Such boredom is not usually a sign of depression.

However, it is a sign when young people have the opportunity to do things they normally enjoy, but do not want to participate. That is the time to worry. Friends do call around, but they do not want to have anything to do with them. They show no interest in PE at school, although this is usually their favourite lesson. If children and teenagers show a change in their behaviour like this over some weeks, this is a clear warning sign of depression.

Disturbed sleep

This can show itself in a number of ways. Difficulty getting off to sleep, waking in the night, being unable to get back to sleep, and waking much earlier than usual in the morning are quite common. Persistent, unhappy and troubling dreams are less common but may occur. So may sleep-walking and sleep-talking, but these are even less common.

How does one know if a child is getting enough sleep? Tiredness and lack of energy during the day are signs of this. On the other hand, the fact that a child will not go to sleep when parents think he or she should is not necessarily a sign of depression, or, indeed, of anything at all being wrong with the child. Some children and teenagers do genuinely have less need for sleep than most. The child who has a lot of energy during the day is probably getting enough sleep, although parents might wish they saw less of him or her in the late evenings!

Changes in appetite

Some children with depression become very picky and go off their food. Others turn to food for comfort and eat far more than is healthy. Either way, if there is a persistent change in attitude towards food, this is a worrying sign.

Dieting is common, especially in teenage girls, but is not itself a sign of depression. It is the girl who does not enjoy food who is much more likely to be depressed. And most girls who diet feel exactly the opposite about their food.

However, dieting may express that a girl is unhappy with the way that she looks and this may well be a reflection of her generally depressed view of herself.

If a girl diets to an excessive degree because she is preoccupied with her appearance when she is, in fact, of perfectly normal weight, or even underweight, then she is probably suffering from anorexia or is likely to do so. That is also a cause of great concern. Some girls (and occasionally boys) with anorexia also show signs of depression, but this is not usually the case.

Suicidal thoughts or behaviour

Without doubt, this is the most worrying of all the signs of depression, and rightly so. Every year probably something like one in a hundred 12- to 16-year-olds makes a suicide attempt. (That will mean 10 students in a secondary school with about 1000 students on the roll.) About one in seven deaths in the 15- to 19 year age group is due to suicide. Fortunately, both suicide and attempted suicide are very much less common under the age of 13 or 14 years, but they do occur.

Not all children who have suicidal ideas are depressed. Fleeting thoughts that life is not worth living are really quite common in the young without depression. A child who stamps a foot when denied a favourite television programme, and says 'All right, I'll kill myself' may just be copying behaviour seen on some other television programme. And if the child is out playing with friends half an hour later, this is likely to be the case. Furthermore, some children who make suicide attempts, or even succeed in taking their own lives, are not depressed. They may be angry and impulsive youngsters or perfectionists fearful of failure and faced by an ordeal that they think may be beyond them. But there is no doubt that depression is an important underlying factor in many suicide attempts. Any indication of suicidal intention must be taken very seriously.

Signs of depression

9

Recognising that a youngster has persistent suicidal thoughts is often not an easy matter. Numerous surveys have revealed that parents are usually quite unaware of whether their teenage children have these thoughts, and it is not at all uncommon for them to be able to cover up from their parents when they have actually made a suicide attempt. Obviously, if children show depression in the other ways described here, it is important to consider the possibility that they may have suicidal ideas. Remarks by a child or a teenager that they are feeling hopeless or that life is not worth living should be taken seriously. Indeed, persistent hopelessness about the future and a view of the future as bleak and unpleasurable are further signs of depression.

With younger children their play may reveal how they are feeling. Play with dolls that constantly repeats themes of separation from parents, dangerous or reckless play, destructive play, and play that constantly involves life-endangering themes – all these may indicate that even quite a young child of 6 or 7 has suicidal ideas.

Of course a lot of children, especially boys, will be taken up with fantasy figures like Superman, whose life is constantly in danger, and when deciding if a boy's play is really a sign of depression one needs to think about whether there are other signs as well.

It is difficult for parents and teachers to accept that a teenager may be having suicidal ideas. For parents, particularly those who have themselves had suicidal ideas and who are under stress, the additional load of such thoughts in their child may be just too much to bear. For a teacher stressed by demands made, for example, by the National Curriculum and perhaps other problems at home, the thought that a student might be suicidal creates possible responsibilities for action it might be easier not to take. For a friend, there will be the guilt of not recognising a best friend's distress. Yet the recognition of suicidal thoughts in a depressed teenager may be a life-saving achievement.

Friends of a suicidal teenager will find themselves in a difficult position if their friend confides their suicidal wishes but swears them to secrecy. Young people sometimes feel that they are the only ones who understand their friend and try to keep things secret. But this is an unfair burden – and possibly a dangerous one. Friends will be doing their best for their depressed friend by letting responsible adults know and not keeping the secret.

Sometimes friends are not aware:

When Sue, at 15 years old, attempted suicide by taking an overdose, her best friend was stunned. 'I didn't know anything was wrong with her. Yes, I realised she had been a bit weepy and unhappy recently, but I just put it down to "that time of the month". When the class heard that she'd tried to kill herself they were freaked out. Some of them reacted by calling her a nutter and then not wanting anything to do with her. But a few of us were really tearful because we were frightened that we would end up doing the same thing, and maybe no one would succeed in stopping us.'

Teachers need to be aware of the copycat effect that sometimes arises following a pupil's attempted or successful suicide. Other pupils' anxieties and fears of not being able to cope can be stirred up by the event, and some may be tempted to turn to self-harm too. Discussions in the classroom can be helpful. It is useful to allow time for each child to express feelings about what has happened, about the loss of a school friend and whether they feel guilty that they could, somehow, have stopped it. One should be particularly sensitive with more vulnerable children who may be experiencing similar feelings and anxieties.

Negative thoughts

It has been suggested that people who are depressed have what have been called 'negative automatic thoughts'. These are thoughts that are 'negative' because they are linked with unpleasant feelings, such as feeling sad or bad about oneself. And are 'automatic' because they seem to just pop into people's heads. For example, if someone makes a mistake (as we all do, of course), the thought might pop up: 'everything I do is wrong' or 'if I can't do it 100% right, there's no point in doing it at all'. Then, feelings of being useless and hopeless may follow. Parents, teachers or friends can help by pointing out, for instance, that we all make mistakes and no one is perfect.

Self-blame

Depressed children and teenagers sometimes take the troubles of their families, their friends and even the world in general on their own shoulders. They may be perfectionists and have set very high standards for themselves. They may blame themselves for arguments their parents have, for the separation of their parents, for an illness in a brother or sister. Reassurance that they are not responsible may fail to convince them.

Self-blame is not one of the more common signs of depression in children and teenagers, but it does occur. Again, talking with them about the stressful events in their lives may reveal these ideas. With younger children their playing or drawings may show how badly they feel about their lives, and how they feel they deserve to be punished for things they have not done.

More commonly, there is a loss of self-esteem. The child or youngster just has a very poor view of him- or herself. Low self-esteem and depression are very closely linked, although they are not identical. Occasionally, a child may have one without the other.

Other signs

In thinking about whether a child or teenager is depressed, the presence of any of the problems described here should be regarded as a warning sign. But there are other issues to bear in mind. Has there been a change in the child's normal behaviour? A child who is happy not to see friends more than occasionally is different from a sociable child who gradually stops wanting to see friends. How is the child's everyday life affected? The child who is functioning really well despite the presence of these problems is less a cause for concern than a child who is, for example, unable to do schoolwork, losing weight or missing school activities.

Is the child's 'depression' a normal response to a recent serious loss? If father has just left home, or a teenage girl has broken off a relationship with a long-standing boyfriend, many of the above problems may be present for several weeks, and that would be quite normal. But if the child's mood remains constantly depressed for longer, this is a real cause for concern.

It is not always easy to distinguish depression from understandable distress. But in some ways it is not all that important to do so. If a child or teenager remains depressed or distressed, whatever you like to call it, over several weeks, there is reason to be worried and to want to do something about it. Suicidal thoughts and suicidal behaviour are a major cause for concern, whatever one calls the problem underlying them, and however severe or apparently trivial the disappointment or loss the child has experienced.

Psychotic depression

If this were a book about depression in adults, we would need to spend some time on this subject. Fortunately, psychotic depressive illnesses are rare in children and adolescents under the age of 16 years, but they do very occasionally occur, so we must mention them briefly. Nearly all teenagers show mood swings to some degree, but some get very depressed and then in other phases are unusually cheerful, talkative and energetic. In a small proportion of these, very worrying changes occur.

The main special features are delusions (false ideas that cannot be changed even though they are obviously wrong) and hallucinations (usually hearing voices or seeing things that are not there). These psychotic symptoms are often accompanied by a dramatic slowing up of movement and speech. The child may also refuse, or not be able, to eat. Sometimes these psychotic episodes alternate with unusually cheerful moods of over-excitement and over-talkativeness. This is called a bipolar disorder. However, such 'hypomanic' episodes may not occur, and there may just be repeated episodes of severe depression. The disorder is then called unipolar.

Treatment involves counselling and support, medication, and, very, very occasionally, electroconvulsive therapy.

It needs to be emphasised that this type of problem is very rare indeed in those under 16 years of age. When it does occur, however, it always needs specialist treatment.

Chronic fatigue

Persistent tiredness and lack of energy are important signs of depression. When these are the most prominent problems, someone may diagnose the child or teenager as having myalgic encephalo-myelitis (MF) or post-viral fatigue syndrome. This form of illness sometimes follows a viral or flu-like illness. The child shows extreme fatigue after exercise, for example. The problem may be prolonged, lasting weeks or even months. The disorder has much in common with depression – in particular, it often has both physical and psychological components. It usually responds well to gentle rehabilitation, and this can sometimes best be provided by a specialist child and adolescent mental health team. Parents of children with chronic fatigue syndrome or ME may feel that the mental health team does not take the physical component of their child's problem sufficiently seriously because they are using entirely a psychological approach. In fact, most mental health professionals do accept there is a physical contribution to chronic fatigue syndrome; they also know that the best way to produce improvement is to concentrate on gradual increase in exercise.

Associated problems

Children and young people who are depressed often have other mental health problems and these may be very prominent, so that the depression is masked by them unless it is thought about. The most common associated problem is excessive anxiety and worrying. Indeed, these are so commonly associated that some people think they are part of the same condition. Anxiety is often focused on separation from parents, illnesses or possible death in parents who are quite healthy, particular lessons in school, examinations, losing friends – the list is endless.

Another set of problems commonly linked to depression is difficult, aggressive behaviour. Children and young people who are disobedient, rebellious, verbally and sometimes physically abusive may also be depressed. It is difficult to talk to them about depression because they want to keep their veneer of toughness, but it is sometimes possible.

When children are very troublesome, it is always worthwhile asking oneself if they are not also very unhappy. Just sometimes, showing a difficult child that one has recognised how sad he or she is may provide the first opportunity for real lines of communication to be established.

Another commonly linked set of problems are the eating disorders, especially anorexia nervosa in girls, and very occasionally in boys. Persistent dieting behaviour may be only part of their difficulties.

Finally, and often overlooked because such children are often seen as beyond help, is the link between heavy alcohol or drug consumption and depression. It is surprising to some people that the average weekly consumption of alcohol in 11-year-old boys is six units, and in 15-year-old boys is seven units, the equivalent of three and a half pints of beer. Quite a few drink much more than this. The rate increases quite sharply with age. Young people who drink heavily or who take drugs may get depressed because they run into financial problems and cannot afford the habits they have developed. The effects of misusing alcohol and other substances can often produce depression in themselves. Alternatively, some teenagers develop a drug or alcohol habit because they are seriously depressed and find that drink or drugs help to remove intolerable black moods. Either way, the teenager who is depressed and who also has a drink or drug problem is in trouble and will need help.

3 How common is depression in children and young people?

About 2 in 100 children under the age of 12 are depressed to the extent that they would benefit from seeing a specialist child psychiatrist. However, about another 4 or 5 in every 100 children of this age show significant distress and some of these

could be described as on the edge of depression. The rate goes up with age, so that about 5 in 100 teenagers are seriously depressed, and at least twice that number show significant distress. These figures apply to children living in stable, settled populations in reasonably good social circumstances. In troubled, inner-city areas with high rates of broken homes, poor community support and high crime rates, the level of depression may be twice the figures we have quoted. About 6 in every 100 000 15- to 19-year-old boys and 1 to 2 per 100 000 girls die by suicide each year in the UK. The rates are much lower in 10- to 14-year-old children, and under 10 years suicide is very rare. Attempted suicide is much more frequent, especially in girls, and as many as 2 or 3 girls in every 100 make a suicide attempt at some time during their teenage years. Usually they take tablets. The seriousness of attempts varies a good deal.

These figures relating to depression and suicide mean that in a secondary school in a reasonably settled area, with 1000 children on the roll, about 50 children will be depressed in any one year. In a primary school with about 400 children on the roll in an inner-city area, about 8 children will be seriously depressed, and double that number will be significantly distressed. Other children in these schools, and often quite a lot of them, will have problems such as disruptive behaviour and learning difficulties.

Various factors affect the rates of depression, and these are discussed under separate headings below.

Differences between girls and boys

Before puberty, boys and girls suffer depression to a roughly equal degree. After puberty the rate in girls is higher, so that by 15 or 16 years, it is twice as high as in boys. There could be physical, perhaps glandular or genetic reasons for this. It is rather more likely that girls respond to stress with depressive reactions more often than boys do, because they are more emotionally involved in relationships and in other aspects of their lives.

Ethnic differences

There are no clear-cut differences between ethnic groups. In some developing countries, children and young people are more likely to show physical symptoms when they are depressed than do those living in the more economically developed countries.

Poverty

Poverty and poor social conditions are not, in themselves, causes of depression. However, children living in families where poor home conditions create stress are more likely to be depressed. Parents bringing up their children in circumstances in which they do not know how they are going to get through the week without getting further into debt understandably have difficulty helping their children through the inevitable stresses and disappointments that life brings.

Changes over time

Are children more likely to be depressed now than used to be the case 30 or 40 years ago? Research findings suggest the changes have not been marked, but there may have been a rise in the rate of depression. Rates of attempted suicides admitted to hospital among young people, however, went down in the early 1980s, although they are still much too high. Rates of suicide have been stable for some years, except for a rise in rates for 15- to 19-year-old boys in the 1980s and early 1990s that now seems to have stopped. The rise may well have been because of an increase in alcohol consumption and drug use in youngsters of this age at that time.

4 What causes depression in children and young people?

Depression in a child does not usually have just one cause. It is useful to think of two broad groups of causes. Like a plant, depression grows because a particular seed (perhaps psychological, such as a loss, or perhaps physical, such as a viral infection) has been planted in soil that is good for growth. The child's genes or inherited characteristics, the child's personality and the child's early experiences can be seen together as the soil in which the seed is planted. Just as both seed and soil are necessary for plant growth (you won't get much plant unless you have both of these), so when we look at depression we need to look at both the seeds – the triggering events – and the nature of the child at the time these events occur. It would be meaningless to say that one or the other is the cause: both are necessary. Let us look first at the triggers.

Losses, disappointments and stresses

Loss is an essential part of ordinary growth and development. In fact, it can often be the spur to change and psychological maturity. As we move on to the next stage of life, we have to lose something of the current stage. If we do not let go, we cannot move on. For a child, going to school may be exciting, stimulating and open up new social relationships, but it also entails the loss of the all-day familiarity of home, or closeness to parents. Similar losses occur throughout our lives: becoming a sexual teenager, for example, entails loss of childishness.

What helps with all these losses is the belief that there are secure, trusting relationships to turn to. If the child (or adult for that matter) feels basically confident and hopeful in relationships, losses in the 'real', external world are coped with in an optimistic manner.

We all become distressed and some of us become depressed when faced with significant losses and disappointments. Children are no exception. Furthermore, we are all aware that the degree of distress we experience in relation to a loss depends on the emotional significance to us of the person involved. Again, the same is true for children and young people, but, especially with younger children, it may be difficult to know how significant a loss has been.

All the factors below, and quite possibly others, will affect the significance of the loss to the child. A parent or teacher may be surprised at the extent of upset a loss produces in a child because they have not appreciated the importance of one or more of these issues. For the same reason, parents and teachers may be surprised how apparently unscathed the child is by a loss that seemed likely to be devastating.

Let us take just as an example why a child might be more or less upset at losing a friend.

Why has the friend been lost?

If she or he has had a serious illness and died, this will obviously give a different meaning to the loss than if the child has moved away to another school or neighbourhood, or there has been an argument between the two children.

How close is the relationship?

Did the two children do everything together, or was this a friendship just based on an occasional contact?

How many other friends does the child have?

The child whose only friend has moved away is in a different position from a child who has five or six other children with whom she or he is friendly.

Was there a sexual component to the relationship?

It is going to be more difficult for a teenager to lose a friendship in which there was some degree of physical attraction and, perhaps, a physical relationship.

Is there any 'unfinished business' in the relationship?

For example, did the children have the opportunity to say goodbye to each other? Or did the child find the friend had disappeared when she or he returned to school at the beginning of a new term, maybe because the friend had moved to another town during the school holidays? Were there any unresolved arguments when the children last saw each other? If so, perhaps the child had a fantasy that the friend went away because she or he was angry.

What, if any, opportunity will there be for contact in the future?

Are the two going to write to each other or speak on the phone? Would that help the child cope with the loss?

Other triggers

When a child becomes depressed beyond a degree that one might call normal distress, it is usually fairly obvious what the trigger is. Sometimes, however, it is unclear, and the following list of factors that have been known to act as triggers may be helpful:

- losses – of a parent (through separation or death), a brother or sister, a grandparent or other relative, a friend, an acquaintance, a pet
- disappointments – not going to the school they wanted on school transfer, failing an examination, not doing as well as they hoped in some out-of-school activity (e.g. athletics, ballet, piano), not being able to get to some exciting event, such as a wedding, birthday party, disco
- stresses – arguments in the family (between parents, with one or both parents, with brothers or sisters), pressure to do

---

better at school, a difficult examination, an admission to hospital (or, more importantly, several admissions), bullying at school, violence in the neighbourhood, perhaps related to racism, a physical or mental illness in the child or in someone close to the child

• abuse – clearly, if a child is being violently treated, pressured into unwanted sexual activity, or is being 'put down' or scapegoated a good deal of the time, this is going to act as a serious stress; children react in a variety of ways, of which depression is certainly one

• physical events – a flu-like illness, glandular fever or some other physical illness, an epileptic fit or series of fits.

We have already seen how the same trigger, such as the loss of a friend, can have very different effects in different children. There are three other points that need to be made about triggers.

First, as Claudius in Hamlet said, 'When sorrows come, they come not single spies, but in battalions'. The more triggers a child is experiencing, the more he or she is likely to become depressed.

Second, when a physical stress occurs, it is sometimes difficult to know whether the depression is caused by physical infection or injury, by the stress of being ill and perhaps being admitted to hospital, or by the worried reactions of parents and family or even perhaps by doctors and nurses creating unnecessary anxiety about symptoms.

Third, and this is more complicated, a child or youngster who is already depressed can create a stress that then misleadingly looks as though it is causing the depression when, in fact, the situation should be looked at the other way around. For example, a depressed child may have difficulties concentrating on school work and therefore fail an important examination. Everyone may think the failure has caused the depression, but this would be misleading.

Brothers and sisters

When a child or adolescent is depressed, she or he usually becomes the focus of attention, and other members of the family are often ignored. It is easy to forget the existence of brothers and sisters. Yet some research has shown that if a child is depressed and there are brothers and sisters, more than one in three of them will also be depressed. They need attention too. Indeed, in considering them in addition, the reasons for the first child's depression may become apparent, and ways of helping may become more obvious.

Vulnerability

So much for triggers, or seeds of depression. What about the nature and temperament of the child – the soil into which the seed falls?

Genes and chromosomes

Parents who have had depressive illnesses themselves are, sadly, more likely to have children with depression. That does not mean that all children of parents with depression get depressed too. In fact, most do not, but they do have an increased tendency to do so. Now this could be, and probably partly is, because a depressed parent almost inevitably creates a somewhat stressful environment for the child. A mother who is absorbed with depressed thoughts about the future and feels terrible is going to find it more difficult to provide her child with the necessary warmth, affection and control. She is also going to pass on half her genes. Genes are long strands of protein (DNA) present in every human cell from the time sperm enters the egg and we are conceived. They dictate whether we are going to be taller or shorter than most people, whether we will develop one of a hundred or more rare diseases such as cystic fibrosis, or less rare diseases such as Alzheimer's disease in old age. Perhaps genes also have some effect on whether we have an increased likelihood of becoming depressed. Most experts think they do.

Some people think that unless you are born with a particular characteristic, it cannot be inherited, but that cannot be right. After all, puberty occurs around about the ages of 10 to 15 years because we are programmed by our genes that way, not because of events that happen to us. It is quite possible that, at least in some people, depression is partly genetically caused.

There is now a reasonable amount of information from twin studies and from studies of families suggesting that this is also the case for some children. But it will probably only be in occasional cases that genes are the most important cause.

In those cases where genes are important, how do they exert their effects? They affect the personality (see below), but they may also alter the way the brain functions in response to stress. A great deal of work has been undertaken to see if chemicals (neurotransmitters) that operate in the brain and the

passage of messages between nerve cells are affected in depression. Other work has been undertaken with hormones, particularly steroid hormones that are known to be affected by stress. So far, no conclusive results have appeared, and the role of biochemical factors and glandular secretions in causing childhood depression remains uncertain.

Temperament and personality

One way in which genes can increase the chances of a child becoming depressed is by their effect on moulding the child's personality. As described earlier, the child is born with a given temperament, and this will affect how the care of the parent is experienced by the child, which will in turn affect the quality of care. For instance, a quiet baby with regular body functions such as sleep and feeding will be quite a different baby to care for than a noisy baby who is difficult to satisfy and wakes and feeds irregularly.

If mothers or fathers are anxious, depressed or unsure of themselves, they may not find a way of dealing with the baby that works for them. On the other hand, they may be experienced parents with adequate supports, and rise to the challenge of the more difficult baby in order to help the child feel more secure in the early days.

This early pattern of relating may have longer-term effects in later life. Children who feel understood and in tune with their environment will have a greater inner security and trust that things will work out in the long run. Those who feel the world is at odds with their own needs could well become more pessimistic.

In later years, as they move into school, some children remain easily upset, cry readily and are discouraged by minor disappointments. Such children may be particularly likely to become depressed, and, even more unfortunately, they may in fact create the circumstances that are likely to produce depression. So, for example, a child with this type of personality can attract bullying at school and thus can, in a sense, be responsible for one of the stresses that can act as a trigger for depression.

This is an example of what is now called 'gene–environment interaction', in which the features of a child's personality cause problems for the child, thus creating further stress for an individual who is poorly equipped to deal with it. Many other examples could be given of this type of interaction.

Earlier experiences

As we have already suggested, children who are depressed have low self-esteem and a negative view of their past experience. Sadly, many children have every right to consider their past experiences disastrous. Children who have been physically or sexually abused, sometimes on a frequent and regular basis, fall into this category. If they have not been made depressed by their experiences, they are nevertheless prone to depression as they move into adolescence. Children whose early years have been lived under a cloud of physical or mental illness in the family, perhaps an alcohol problem in their father or a depressive illness in their mother, may have been sensitised to further stress. Unexpected early separations, such as an emergency admission to hospital, may also have made the child vulnerable, so that even a minor further separation may reactivate a worry that is always just below the surface.

Other long-lasting difficulties

Some children suffer from long-lasting difficulties that make them particularly prone to depression. Thus, children with chronic physical disorders such as diabetes, cystic fibrosis, asthma and, more especially, epilepsy and cerebral palsy, are at slightly greater risk. The same is true for children with learning difficulties at school. It should be emphasised that most children with these long-lasting difficulties will not be depressed, but they are at slightly greater risk.

Coping skills and protective factors

When a child has to face a disappointment or a stress, she or he is not just a passive individual taking what comes without the ability to do anything about it. Children and teenagers respond actively to bad experiences in order to try to master and overcome them. These 'coping skills' help to explain why some children do not become depressed, even though faced with terrible adversity. Similarly, some children faced with adversity have positive things going for them in their environment, and if these protective factors are present, they lower the risk of depression. Helpful coping skills include the ability to confide worries to friends and family members, and the capacity to deal with one problem at a time rather than be overwhelmed by a mass of difficulties. Children who have a particularly good relationship with one or both parents, who have someone outside the immediate family, such as a grandparent, in whom they can confide, who have some special skills or a talent for athletics or artistic ability – all are less likely to develop depression when stressful circumstances strike. Just as some children have personalities that make them vulnerable to depression, so others have optimistic personalities that mean that they are more likely to survive troubling times without becoming depressed.

The protective factors and coping skills enjoyed by children and teenagers are important because they sometimes give clues as to how we can best help them under stress. Reinforcing natural strengths is often a better idea than trying to invent completely new methods of treatment to deal with weaknesses.

Understanding the causes of depression is quite complicated if we try to produce a scheme that fits all children. The diagram below is an attempt to bring all these factors together. You will see how some factors push the young person towards more serious depression, while others enhance resistance. But, of course, no diagram can do justice to the richness involved in the life of any one particular child.

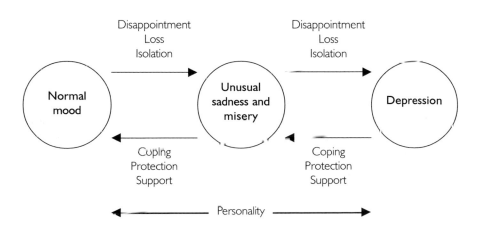

5　Helping a depressed child – what you (parents, teachers, children) can do

As the poet John Donne said, 'no man is an island' – we all need people. But when we are sad, distressed or unhappy, we need other people even more – even if we think we do not!

There is a great deal that can be done by parents, teachers and others to help depressed children, and on page 37 we provide action sheets for guidance.

Listening

Listening to children sounds so simple and obvious, but sometimes it is the quality of the listening that counts more than anything. It is, in fact, rather difficult to listen to children (or people generally) in distress. There are many reasons why children do not get heard in everyday life. For example, in school, they may be overlooked if:

- they are quiet and withdrawn
- the class is too big and troublesome
- teachers are too tired or worried themselves.

Both parents and teachers may find themselves overlooking depressed children if:

- they are too wrapped up in their own problems (perhaps death of a relative or friend, marriage problems, how to make ends meet)
- they feel helpless and useless in the face of someone else's despair
- they are just too busy
- it is too upsetting to think about.

So, it is important to look at yourself, to ask whether you are hearing children's distress and to think about what could be done to help you to listen better. Caring for ourselves enables us to care for our children. As a parent, are you depressed yourself? Support, help, advice and even treatment for parents are important aspects of helping children. It is important not to feel that a child's problems are all your fault, as this, too, may be a block to your listening in a positive way.

Teachers and other professionals may need to look at their practice. Are you overworked – and who is not? Do you need support to think about the multitude of problems presenting in everyday situations? Regular supervision or discussion with someone outside the busy work setting can really help to pick up problems that may otherwise be overlooked.

Aspects of listening

Try listening with the heart and not just the ears. Imagine the child's distress by relating it (in your mind only) to periods of distress in your own life.

Do not belittle the child's unhappiness. Behind every attention-seeker is a real problem that perhaps the child needs to dramatise in order to ensure an audience. If the child does not feel you are taking the problem seriously, you run the risk of the child heightening the drama, and perhaps acting in a self-destructive way.

As a parent, if you think your child is attention-seeking, you need to ask why she or he needs so much attention. What is it that this child is trying to draw attention to?

Time

- Give time to listen properly
- Minimise external distractions
- Unplug or switch off the telephone
- Find a private, secluded room
- Do not allow interruptions – these will make the child feel that the problem is just a burden for you and that you do not, after all, have the time and patience to listen properly.

Listening

- Do not recount your own worries or upset the child
- Do not tell stories about other people's problems
- Let the child see that you take the problems and worries seriously, however trivial you may find them
- Do not attempt to cheer the child up with phrases like 'come on now, it's not the end of the world' or 'it may never happen' – it may just feel like the end of the world to this child, since she or he feels that 'it' has already happened
- Do not blame the child.

Reflect back

Children feel heard and understood if you summarise what they have said by repeating or putting what they have said in another way. Sometimes it may be necessary to comment on how they look, if they find it difficult to verbalise (e.g. 'you do look upset' or 'I can see how difficult it is to talk about this').

Drawing or play

Younger children may find it too hard to talk about their feelings. It can be suggested that they draw whatever it is they are feeling or are worried about. They may express themselves with the help of toys, such as families of dolls and a dolls' house, puppets or toy animals.

Offer hope

Given that despair and hopelessness are features of depression it is useful to think of keeping hope alive for the child. It may help to suggest:

- that these feelings will eventually pass
- that there are ways they can be helped, either through talking or by referral to specialists.

Offer help to challenge negative thought patterns

Negative thought patterns (i.e. always seeing the worst) are a common feature of depression. For example, after a school-time dispute with a playmate, the child might say 'See, no one likes me – I have no friends'. It would help for parents and teachers to examine the 'evidence' of this with the child. 'Didn't Amy ask you to her party last week?'; 'When I picked you up from school John and Sally said goodbye to you'. It helps to ask the child to try to think about similar situations and provide their own 'evidence' too.

Offer practical help

If it is possible to change whatever it was that brought about the depression, it should be changed. There may also be practical things that will help, such as arranging for friends to come round, or planning and going on an outing.

However, let's be realistic: by no means everything that brings about a child's depression can be changed. Maybe parents have separated; father has another family and has lost interest in his first children. Maybe mother has a drink problem she is finding hard to beat. Perhaps the child has a serious physical illness that is chronic, or even progressing. When these problems will not go away, and the child's mood persists, all the other ways of helping – listening, keeping up the support, sharing feelings and so on – become even more important.

But, do not forget, some problems you think cannot go away may be helped to disappear. Not so long ago, for example, many schoolteachers felt helpless in the face of bullying. They said there was nothing they could do – 'boys will be boys' – and girls can be pretty horrible to each other too. But now all schools are expected to have an anti-bullying policy, and much more is being done to prevent this unpleasant aspect of school life.

Keep up the support

Let children know that, until they are feeling better, you are available to them whenever they want to talk to you.

Keep in touch

Do not allow the child to withdraw. This is difficult to achieve without being intrusive. We all know the sullen, uncommunicative teenager who insists that things are all right and tells you to go away. However, you should:

- keep an eye open, and keep watch at a distance, if that is all they will permit
- persist in expressing your concern from time to time
- not allow yourself to be fobbed off
- if worried, take it further (see the action sheets on page 37).

Physical contact

Given possible allegations about sexual abuse involving teachers these days, there is much concern about whether physical contact is appropriate or not. This is a great pity because ordinary human empathy and spontaneity could be lost. Sometimes depressed and distressed children need an adult to put an arm around them, to give comfort. It would be sad for this to be denied them. Respond naturally. If a child draws away, do not insist, but continue to talk.

Teachers will be aware of the dangers of having comforting physical contact misinterpreted. This is much less likely to happen if the contact is limited, as it should be, to a briefly held hand contact, a pat on the back or an arm on the shoulder. Misunderstanding is also less likely to occur if there are other people around and they know that you are attempting to support the child in question.

Confidentiality

Sometimes children will tell a trusted adult, outside their family, of their depression (or suicidal feelings) and insist that this remains a secret. This poses quite a dilemma. How much should the confidentiality be respected; to what extent do parents have a right to know about their child's difficulties? The answer is that parents do have the right to know. And if the situation is severe (as outlined at the start of this chapter), or if the child is at risk of suicide, there is a duty to inform parents.

However, in less worrying situations, it may be possible for, say, a teacher to see a child a few times in order to understand the problem better. It may be that poor communication with the parents is, in fact, part of the problem.

Confidentiality is going to be more of a problem for a teacher when there is suspected abuse at home, perhaps because of something the child has said. In these cases the teacher should talk with the head teacher and a social worker will need to be contacted.

In other circumstances, a joint meeting with the child and parents to air concerns is nearly always helpful.

Seeking professional help

It is important to know, however, when the techniques above are not sufficient and the child needs specialist help. Professional help should be sought when:

- the depression does not lift after 2 to 3 weeks
- there is interference with daily life
- there is severe disturbance of sleep and eating patterns
- suicidal thoughts or wishes are expressed.

How to get specialist help

Help for problems mainly at home

If the problems are occurring mainly at home and do not improve, then the parents' first port of call should be the family doctor. Most family doctors nowadays see emotional problems in children and teenagers as part of their job, although obviously some are going to be more interested than others (that is true of all professionals). Your doctor will, of course, want to see your child and have a chat with him or her, either with you, separately or all together. If your child does not want to go to the doctor (and this is not at all unusual), then you, the parent or parents, should go anyway to discuss the situation. You may be in need of help so that you continue to cope, and your doctor may be able to provide assistance here.

Anyway, after seeing you and your child, the doctor will listen, give advice and support. Often there will be a need for further appointments to see how the problem is progressing. If, after several weeks, the problem is no better or even seems to be getting worse, then your doctor will probably suggest a referral to the local child and family psychiatric clinic (discussed in the next chapter). This may have been suggested earlier if the problem is severe. If your doctor does not suggest a referral, then you can suggest one yourself.

Help for problems mainly at school

Once a problem in school has been identified by teachers, parents, or the teenager himself or herself, there needs to be a get-together with everyone (and that 'everyone' includes the child) involved to decide what to do. It will often be helpful for the child to be present from the beginning. Sharing of information in this situation is nearly always going to be useful. If whatever is decided does not prove helpful enough, then a referral should be made, either to the child and family psychiatric clinic, or, if the problem is mainly to do with learning difficulties or behaviour in the classroom, to the educational psychologist attached to the school.

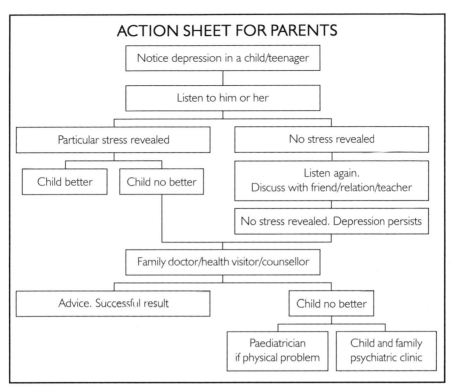

ACTION SHEET FOR PARENTS

Notice depression in a child/teenager

Listen to him or her

Particular stress revealed

No stress revealed

Child better

Child no better

Listen again.
Discuss with friend/relation/teacher

No stress revealed. Depression persists

Family doctor/health visitor/counsellor

Advice. Successful result

Child no better

Paediatrician
if physical problem

Child and family
psychiatric clinic

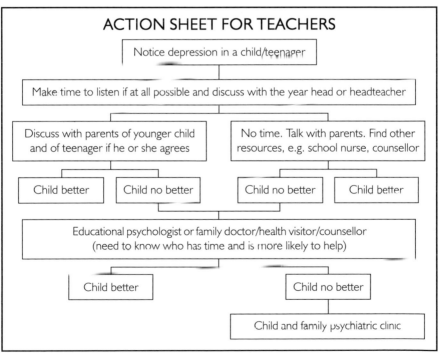

ACTION SHEET FOR TEACHERS

Notice depression in a child/teenager

Make time to listen if at all possible and discuss with the year head or headteacher

Discuss with parents of younger child
and of teenager if he or she agrees

No time. Talk with parents. Find other
resources, e.g. school nurse, counsellor

Child better

Child no better

Child no better

Child better

Educational psychologist or family doctor/health visitor/counsellor
(need to know who has time and is more likely to help)

Child better

Child no better

Child and family psychiatric clinic

---

6 The child and adolescent mental health clinic

Services for child and adolescent mental health problems have different names. They may be called, for example, 'child and adolescent mental health clinic', 'family consultation clinic', 'child guidance clinic' or 'young people's clinic'. Some are situated in hospitals, while others are attached to health centres or are on school premises.

Who works in these clinics?

In most clinics there will be a number of different child and adolescent mental health professionals. Usually there will be at least one psychologist, psychiatrist, nurse and social worker. There may also be a child psychotherapist and/or a family therapist. These professionals differ in their training and backgrounds. But despite these differences, their skills overlap a good deal. They will all have had training in how to assess emotional problems and in counselling of parents and children. They will all have well-developed skills in listening and in picking up clues about what might be going wrong by careful observation. Often they will also be skilled in a number of different types of treatment, including psychotherapy with individual children and parents, setting up behavioural programmes and family therapy.

As well as these shared skills, they will all have special responsibilities and interests. Psychologists often have special skills in assessing learning difficulties and in devising behavioural programmes such as those described in the section 'Cognitive behavioural therapy' below. Child psychiatric nurses will have a background in mental health nursing and will often be particularly skilled in behavioural management and in working with families in the home. The child and adolescent psychiatrist, who is a qualified doctor, combines knowledge of the emotional and behavioural problems of children and young people with a medical background. Child psychotherapists have had a long training in individual child psychotherapy and will have special skills in understanding the 'internal world' of the child. Social workers are generally known for their role in child protection, and this is part of their work, but they will mainly be concerned with improving relationships in the family. They also have special knowledge of the benefits system that may be helpful. Family therapists specialise in observation of the way family members interact together and in trying to intervene helpfully as a result of their observations. There may also be other therapists such as art or music therapists, or health professionals called mental health workers.

How do the people at the clinic work?

First, there may be a waiting time, and this is likely to be between 1 and 3 months. However, most clinics have an emergency procedure for cases that clearly cannot wait. To save time, the clinic may ask you to provide some information on a questionnaire before you arrive. They may also ask permission to contact your child's school, so that by the time of your appointment, the staff have some idea about your child's progress and behaviour in school.

Often families are worried by the first appointment letter, which requests the attendance of the whole family. They may feel that the clinic is suggesting they are to blame in some way for the child's problems. In fact, clinic staff are trained to understand and not to blame. It is very helpful to have the whole family's views of the current difficulties to help assess the young person and the situations in which the problems occur.

When you arrive, the member or members of the clinic staff who are seeing you, usually one or two people, will introduce themselves and explain how the assessment will be carried out and how long it will take. Some clinics use one-way screens or video equipment, either for training purposes for staff attached to the clinic who are learning, or because it is felt to be a good way to have more than one view of the problem. If it is intended to use either video or a one-way screen, this will be explained to you and your consent will be necessary for its use. You may find this approach too prying and you have every right to withhold consent. However, it can be helpful to those who are trying to understand and help your child and family.

A big difference between the clinic and the general practitioner is the greater amount of time available at the clinic, usually an hour or more. Further, the staff have had special training in listening to children and parents talking about their problems, so they will have greater experience in assessing children and young people who are unhappy and depressed.

Their approach is likely to involve working with the child and family in a collaborative way. They may begin by wishing to see the whole family together and then the child or young person separately, before seeing the parent or parents on their own.

Most professionals working in child and adolescent mental health clinics have a favoured approach. They may, for example, put most emphasis on seeing the whole family or they may mainly work with the child or adolescent alone. Some will be more interested in dealing directly with the symptoms or complaints, and others in what is going on underneath. All will want to spend time listening and trying to understand the predicament in which the child and family find themselves. While, in some circumstances, most professional staff will prescribe or recommend the prescription of tablets, they will probably not want to recommend medication until they know the child better and have explored other possibilities.

Towards the end of the assessment, the member(s) of the clinic staff who have seen you are likely to explain how they see the problem in the first instance and what they suggest for the future. Some families are offered advice on the spot and it is suggested that they return only if problems persist. However, the staff are quite likely to think it would be a good idea to see the child or adolescent on a number of occasions for treatment following the assessment visit. They may, for example, explain that rapid change is not to be expected but they are hopeful that, with treatment, there could be some improvement over the next few weeks or months. They will write to your family doctor or whoever has referred you, giving the results of the assessment. They may wish to be in touch with the school again.

Charles

When Charles was 8 years old he was referred by his family doctor because he had been having stomach-aches and headaches for the past 6 months. As a result of these pains, he had missed school for most of these 6 months. He had been previously seen by a paediatrician, who had done some blood tests, all of which had turned out to be normal. The paediatrician thought the pains were psychological, and had given some advice, but the pains and school absence had persisted.

The psychologist who saw Charles, an only child, and his parents had previously written asking for a school report. His teachers said there wasn't too much they could say about him as he had been absent so much, but, as far as they could see, he was a pleasant, quiet boy who had no problems with the school work, though he had rather few friends. The school expressed concern about his absences, which they had been told had a physical cause and asked to be kept in the picture.

The psychologist saw Charles and his parents together to begin with. She noted that Charles sat very close to his mother and that his father sat a little separately. The psychologist asked the family to explain how they saw the problem and whether they thought coming to the clinic was a good idea. Mrs X immediately began to speak. She said that she had not been at all keen to come to the clinic. She was still pretty convinced the problem was physical. She talked for quite a long time about how 'normal' Charles was and how there was no one in the family who had had nervous trouble. It turned out, however, that since the onset of the pains Charles had really been very easily upset, tearful and sleeping poorly. He was unable to settle to anything, even computer games that he normally enjoyed. The psychologist obtained a full account of the development of the symptoms and of other aspects of the background to the referral. It was, however, difficult for her to bring Mr X or Charles into the conversation. Mr X just said he left this sort of thing to his wife.

The psychologist then saw Charles by himself. He was nervous about being separated from his parents, but eventually allowed them to leave him in the room with the psychologist, who had particular experience in interviewing young children. Charles would not talk to her, but she eventually managed to encourage him to play with some family dolls. The way he played, especially with the female dolls, suggested to her that he was quite an angry boy. She was really unable to draw any other conclusions in this first interview.

She then saw the parents by themselves while Charles was looked after in the waiting area by a receptionist. She asked whether there was anything else the couple wanted to tell her that they had not wanted to say in front of Charles. It seemed as if Mr X might have something to say, but he seemed unable to bring himself to do so. The psychologist said she thought that Charles really was suffering from depression and anxiety and that his pains were somehow linked to these feelings.

Over the next 3 months the psychologist saw the family on several more occasions. She also worked with the school to monitor Charles's attendance there. A mixture of family sessions and individual therapy for Charles proved helpful and gradually Charles's pains became less frequent, he started to see his friends again and his school attendance became much more regular.

Emma

Emma was a 15-year-old girl who was first seen by a child and adolescent psychiatrist 2 days after she had been sent to an accident and emergency department, having swallowed 20 paracetamol tablets. She had had to have a stomach washout, had been very unwell, and had been lucky not to have suffered any permanent damage to her kidneys or liver. When the psychiatrist saw her she was very tearful and upset. She explained to him that she had been feeling low for about 4 months, since she had had an attack of 'flu. Gradually she had become more and more depressed, not wanting to see her friends, hating school, sleeping poorly and being irritable with her parents and her younger sister. She felt people talked about her behind her back. She couldn't get out of her mind an episode about 6 months ago when she had been responsible for another girl being pushed out of her group of friends because of a row over a boy at the neighbouring school.

The psychiatrist saw Emma's parents, who explained that they just didn't know what had been wrong with their daughter. She had been just so irritable over the previous few months that she had made life impossible for everybody. They had not known what to do for the best. Every time they had tried to talk to her she had snapped at them. They were appalled that she had tried to end her life. It turned out that Emma's father had himself been depressed for several months about 6 years ago, but he had not been irritable and it had not occurred to her parents that she might have the same problem. The psychiatrist took a full account of the problem from both Emma and her parents and came to the conclusion that Emma had a depressive illness.

Emma was offered and accepted a course of cognitive–behavioural therapy. The psychological treatment aimed to help her to check on how realistic her thoughts were. She kept a diary noting when she thought people were talking about her and why she had come to this conclusion. However progress was slow and in the clinical review meeting, after the 4th session, the therapist expressed the view that the level of Emma's depression was making it difficult to progress her therapy. The psychiatrist recommended that Emma be given an antidepressant in addition to and alongside the cognitive-behavioural theray. Over the next 4-6 weeks she slowly improved both in her thinking and in her mood and became less irritable and depressed. Although Emma had another bout of depression at university, she remained well for most of the time and was able to lead a very normal and enjoyable life for the rest of her school days and at university.

What types of treatment are provided?

Cognitive–behavioural therapy

Depression can also be seen as a disorder of thinking, and we have already described how some children and teenagers blame themselves when they have not done anything wrong. If we think we have done something wrong in the past, or that the future is hopeless, we may become depressed – our mood follows our thoughts. And if these ideas are false, our mood is inappropriate and undeserved. So, people who use cognitive therapy argue, helping a depressed child or teenager to think differently and more accurately about his or her past, present or future will also help lift the depression.

Although there are certain similarities, this is quite a different approach to that taken by psychoanalytic therapists, who tend to think of inaccurate thoughts and ideas as following mood rather than the other way around.

How do cognitive therapists, and they may be psychologists or psychiatrists, work? First, the child is asked to explain what she or he means by words like 'angry', 'happy', 'worried', 'cheerful', 'sad' and 'depressed', and to give some examples of when she or he recently experienced these. The child is also asked to describe thoughts and ideas at the time of these experiences. Next, she or he is asked to keep a diary of moods and the thoughts accompanying them. Following this, the child is asked to try to make links between thoughts and the moods that go with them. One or two tasks may then be set, and it is suggested that the child will feel happier when the task is accomplished.

The child will face difficult situations. It is suggested that she or he thinks of different solutions and chooses one of them. For example, a boy may be faced with a bully at school and helped to choose whether to tell a teacher, his parents, work out ways of avoiding the bully, talk to other boys about ways of avoiding the bully, and so on. A girl may be helped to examine whether ideas that people are against her or think little of her are accurate, and encouraged to check such ideas against reality. Improved social relationships can be linked to improved mood states.

Specific techniques such as role play with the therapist can sometimes help to make change easier for the child. As time goes on the child is encouraged to challenge previous assumptions that events around him or her have a negative significance. For example, a child may be helped to see that a mother's bad moods are not caused by the child's behaviour, but have all sorts of other reasons. The core of the treatment involves self-monitoring and problem-solving at a conscious level.

Family therapy

So far, we have talked about childhood depression as being a problem located within the child, but this is not always how things are viewed in terms of treatment. Family therapists would want to think about the whole family, not just the person who presents with problems. As we have said above, this is not because the family is felt to be the 'cause' of the problem, but rather because no one member in a family exists in isolation from the others. Family therapists view the problem a child shows as serving a purpose for the family as a whole unit. Thus, a depressed child can be understood only within a set of family relationships, constantly acting upon each other in a circular way. In other words, the problem does not belong to the child, but to the family. The child is showing behaviour in relation to other family members.

> Ian, aged 12 years and an only child, was brought to a clinic by his parents, who were worried and also exasperated by his depression, lack of interest in activities he previously enjoyed, and feelings of hopelessness. His father did most of the talking, explaining how he had tried everything to bring his son out of himself. Ian's mother was silent, but the family therapist felt she was very angry, especially with her husband. It gradually became clear that Ian's father had been made redundant 6 months previously, and was having no success in finding another job. He was spending much more time with Ian.

Previously, Ian's mother had made all the decisions about her son, but now she felt pushed out. She had started to argue with her husband about the way he was taking Ian away from his friends to go fishing and to football matches with him. Ian had then started to say he did not want to go out at all. His father then criticised him, and his mother withdrew more. When the situation became clear to the therapist and the parents it was possible for them to argue less about Ian, and his depression lifted, although it did not disappear completely.

Family therapy takes the form of meetings with the entire family (defined as all those who live at home) and a family therapist. These may be limited to an agreed number of sessions (often six to eight), or may be open-ended, over a longer period. Often they occur at fortnightly intervals in order to permit the family to work on things at home between sessions.

Very often the meetings take place in a large room, one wall of which is a one-way mirror. The family therapist may have a co-worker who will observe the session from behind this mirror-screen, in order to gain an independent perspective on the events taking place within the therapy room.

Sometimes the sessions are videotaped (always with written permission from the parents), so that the therapist can review them at a later stage, perhaps with family members themselves.

Family therapists work through understanding and changing the way family members interact with each other. Very often family trees are drawn during the family sessions, to help clarify just what the family tasks are at this stage of the children's lives. Each stage presents the family members with psychological and relationship tasks to perform. Family difficulties may arise at times of change. Other family members might have their own 'life-cycle issues', which will all interact within the family unit. For example, family life changes when a teenager begins working towards greater independence, and eventually leaves home. The family as a whole is affected. Relationships between the parents will be affected; they have to look to their future as a couple again, as their children leave. Loss may be central to the whole family's functioning, and may be associated with grandparents becoming elderly or dying.

The great advantage of family therapy is that it allows for improved communication, especially when family members have things they find difficult to talk about without help. The therapist will therefore be particularly interested to hear family members who have difficulty in making their thoughts and feelings known.

Family therapy is not interested in 'blame' and not even concerned with causes, but works by understanding just how the family is working together. The whole family is affected by a difficulty, and can in turn affect the resolution of it.

Psychoanalytic psychotherapy

Child psychotherapists take the view that much depression is caused by emotions and thoughts that the child or teenager finds difficult to bring to the surface. The psychotherapist helps the child to do this through play, drawing or discussion. For some children, changes within the family, or the lifting of pressures upon them, are not enough to help them overcome their complex feelings.

Psychotherapy looks not only at problem areas but at the child's whole personality and coping strategies. Appointments are offered at regular intervals, often once a week or occasionally more frequently, in order to develop the therapeutic relationship.

What happens?

Psychotherapy takes place in a private room – always the same room, with the same toys and furniture. The therapist and child meet one to one. The child may be encouraged to find expression in playing with toys or in drawing. Often, however, especially with older children, treatment is entirely through talking.

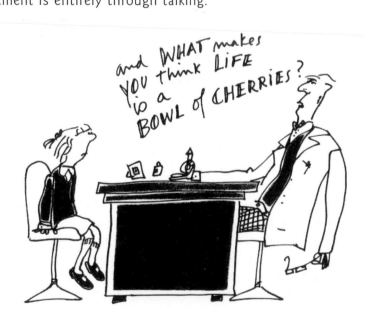

The following examples show how two depressed boys had reacted quite differently to the development of diabetes. Both boys reacted against the diabetic treatment, and would not become involved in planning either a diet or an insulin regime. Both became withdrawn and their school work deteriorated.

> Steven was only interested in sport, both playing it and watching it. His increased activity led to further problems with control of his diabetes. During psychotherapy it emerged that he had great anxieties about the loss of control over his body. He felt that all the injections had damaged his body's ability to hold together – as if his skin was punctured all over and could not hold him in.

> Darren's worries were quite different. He was primarily concerned about feeling different from other people. He had particular difficulty in feeling that he could grow up to be an active and effective man, because he felt that he was so unlike his healthy father.

Once these issues were uncovered and addressed in therapy, both boys were able to participate in control of their diabetes and thus settle down again to ordinary life.

A depressed child will gradually develop a relationship with the therapist through play, drawing or talking. In this way the therapist and child explore together how the child copes with life. The psychotherapist will help the child develop an understanding of his or her feelings, and how these affect behaviour and relationships. This may involve exploring how past experiences and relationships affect the child's ways of coping in the present. The therapist will not suggest solutions to children's difficulties, feeling that it is better for them to strengthen their own ability to reason and work out alternatives for themselves, rather than depend on the therapist. Psychotherapy is a gradual process during which children are allowed to explore their depression. The therapist acknowledges what the child is going through, and this empathy and expression of feeling brings relief. It enables the child to move on, psychologically, to discover new strengths and coping abilities.

In the process of therapy children will experience a whole range of feelings towards the therapist, which is both healthy and expected. This does mean that sometimes a child will become reluctant to come to therapy. It can be hard for parents to continue to bring them and they will need encouragement to help the child to continue to come and express these negative feelings. It is particularly important in depression that angry and aggressive feelings which may arise are brought to the surface. It is a relief to the child to discover that these negative feelings can be tolerated and expressed.

The therapist will always keep family issues in mind, and may work with another professional who will see the parents, and sometimes the family, while the child is in psychotherapy. Sometimes the therapist will do this job him- or herself.

Group therapy

In a small number of clinics, children are sometimes treated together in groups of roughly the same age. They may be mixed in terms of gender, although sometimes they are single-gender groups. There will be one or two therapists present.

The group may be focused on a particular subject, with a set agenda, or be less directive and have an open agenda. Group leaders may direct the children into specific activities, aiming to work on particular issues such as cooperation and sharing, or they may let the children decide on the activity and issues together. Sometimes video equipment is used to help the children observe themselves in order to encourage change. Again, written permission from the parents is necessary.

Such groups usually meet once a week or fortnightly. They may run over a short number of agreed sessions or be more open-ended, depending on the way the group itself develops to decide duration or content.

Physical treatments

Physical treatments are usually less important in children with depression than the 'talking' treatments mentioned above, but they are sometimes helpful and, occasionally, they turn out to be the most important part of treatment.

Medication

When the problems of a child or adolescent are at least moderately severe and do not respond to 'talking' treatments, a doctor, usually a child and adolescent psychiatrist, will consider the possible use of medication. In the UK following the 2005 review of depression in children and young people by the National Institute of Health and Clinical Excellence (NICE), the recommendation is that only specialists in child and adolescent psychiatric disorders should start children or adolescents on antidepressants.

There are two main groups of antidepressant medication. For many years the so-called tricyclic antidepressants, especially amitriptyline and imipramine, have been used with depressed children. During the past 20 years, numerous excellent studies have been carried out with this form of medication. Unfortunately, it is now clear that they are not generally effective in treating depression in children and adolescents, although they sometimes may, on specialist advice and in certain circumstances, be worth trying. They do help symptoms of anxiety and improve sleep, and that can make a difference. They also have occasional side-effects, such as a dry mouth and dizziness when standing up.

Newer forms of antidepressant, the so-called selective serotonin reuptake inhibitors (SSRIs), were introduced in the 1980s. These have fewer side-effects and are generally reckoned to be more effective and safer than the tricyclic antidepressants because of a lower risk of serious harm in the case of an overdose. They do have side-effects, although these are mainly minor. In 2003, British doctors were advised against using SSRIs for depression other than fluoxetine with children and adolescents, because of a lack of evidence that they were effective. Subsequent advice from NICE recommends sertraline or citalopram as second-line alternative treatments (after considering fluoxetine) but only after carefully considered circumstances and only initiated by a specialist doctor in the field. There has also been a concern that they might increase the risk of self-harm in young people who take them. When these antidepressant are prescribed there should be full information about them available to the young person and their parents/carers. The child or teenager should be closely monitored and followed up, in particular in the first few weeks after starting medication or changing doses. Such antidepressant medication treatment should take place alongside appropriate specialist psychosocial care which may include, for example, cognitive–behavioural therapy, family therapy or psychodynamic therapy, and not in isolation. When used selectively, in this way, many child and adolescent psychiatrists think, on the basis of their experience and the evidence to date, that these drugs can be helpful, sometimes very helpful, when serious depression is present. If tablets are prescribed, they need to be taken regularly; it might be 2–3 weeks or more before they start to take effect. If they are effective, they should be continued for around 4–6 months after things have got better.

With both these forms of medication, it is important to make sure tablets are kept well out of the way of a teenager who might be suicidal. Of course, that also applies to tablets taken by other members of the household. It is best to keep all tablets locked away, particularly if there are toddlers around, who may mistake them for sweets.

Another form of medication, lithium carbonate, is used very occasionally in older children and teenagers who have bipolar disorder or psychotic depression (see earlier section on psychotic depression). This medication, which is used to prevent attacks of depression, has to be carefully monitored. The teenager has to have regular blood checks to make sure the level of lithium is kept within certain limits.

Other forms of therapy

There are various other forms of specialist treatment for depression that are used from time to time. For example, there are many other ways in which children can be helped to express their feelings, such as art, drama and music therapies. Hypnosis is another example. Occasionally, dietary treatment, involving the removal of certain additives or foods from the diet, is used.

How is a particular treatment selected?

The treatment the child needs will be chosen for a number of reasons. If there are stresses in school or the home that seem to be at the root of the problem, these will naturally be tackled first. In most cases, as the examples of Charles and Emma show, clinic staff are likely to use a combination of approaches. When the problem is seen mainly as within the child, individual therapy of some type is likely to be the most important part of treatment. Where the problem is thought to be in the way family members interact, then family therapy will have more prominence. Other important considerations include the availability of particular treatment types, and the sort of treatment with which the therapist is most experienced. If parents feel unhappy with the form of treatment they are offered, they should not hesitate to raise the matter with a member of the staff of the clinic or with their own doctor.

7 What happens to depressed children and young people?

What happens to depressed children and young people depends very much on the severity of the problem.

The good news is that distressed and mildly depressed children can be expected to improve over several weeks or months, especially if their problems are recognised, sources of unhappiness are dealt with, and they receive sympathetic help.

On the other hand, follow-up studies suggest that more serious forms of depression in children and adolescents (especially those accompanied by marked interference with daily life and persistent suicidal thoughts) do not fare as well. Perhaps as many as a half will go into adult life with a high likelihood of recurrence and the development of further depressive disorders from time to time.

Sadly, depression when it occurs in a severe form in childhood or the teenage years is often by no means a passing phase. But the good news is that children with even quite serious depression are not at unusual risk of developing other mental disorders such as schizophrenia. All this means that a number of youngsters with depression, once they have been identified and recognised, will need help over months and years. It goes without saying that their parents and any brothers or sisters will also need support. Having a child with severe depression in the family is a major load on family life.

We hope, however, that we have made it clear that there is always much that can be done to help a depressed child or teenager, as well as other members of the family. Most children who are distressed or depressed will, fortunately, improve with time, sympathy, and sometimes more expert help.

Further reading

Burningham, S. (1994) *Young People under Stress: A Parent's Guide*. London: Virago.

Coleman, J. Lyon, J. & Piper, R. (2002) *Teenage Suicide and Self-harm* (2nd edn). Tape Pack. Brighton: Trust for the Study of Adolescents.

Holditch, L. (1997) *Understanding Your 5-Year-Old*. London: Warwick Publishing.

Lask, B. (1985) *Children's Problems: A Parent's Guide to Understanding and Tackling Them*. London: Optima.

National Institute for Health and Clinical Excellence (2005) *Depression in Children and Young People*. London: NICE. Available at www.nice.org.uk/Guidance/CG28

Pearce, J. (1994) *Growth and Development*. London: Thorsons.

Treadwell, P. (1988) *A Parent's Guide to the Problems of Adolescence*. Harmondsworth: Penguin.

Waddell, M. (2005) *Understanding 12–14-Year-Olds*. London: Jessica Kingsley Publishers.

YoungMinds (for address see page 54) produce leaflets and booklets for parents and young people. The following might be of particular interest.

YoungMinds Information Leaflets (for parents)

Children and Young People Get Depressed Too. Available free at www.youngminds.org.uk/publications/leaflets/depressed.php

Worried About a Young Person's Eating Problems? Available free at www.youngminds.org.uk/publications/leaflets/eatingproblems.php

YoungMinds Booklets for Young People

Do you ever feel depressed? Available free at www.youngminds.org.uk/publications/booklets/depressed.php

Worried About Eating Disorders? Available free at www.youngminds.org.uk/publications/booklets/eatingdisorders.php

Useful organisations

Your local library will have details of your nearest child and family psychiatric clinic. Most of these will see self-referrals, although they prefer you to have a letter from your doctor.

All these provide information and advice, and some have helplines. We have given website addresses where we think they are useful, but we cannot take responsibility for their content.

ChildLine
Confidential helpline for children and young people.
Freepost NATN 1111, London E1 6BR
Helpline: 0800 1111 (24-hours, free)
www.childline.org.uk

National Children's Bureau
8 Wakley Street, London EC1V 7QE
Telephone: 020 7843 6000
www.ncb.org.uk
Young people's website. www.youngncb.org.uk

Parentline Plus
Informative website and confidential helpline for parents.
Helpline: 0808 800 2222 (24-hours, free)
Textphone: 0800 783 6783 (for people with speech or hearing impairments, 9.00 am to 5.00 pm, Monday to Friday, free).
www.parentlineplus.org.uk

Royal College of Psychiatrists
No helpline. The College's website has information on depression as well as on emotional problems in young people.
www.rcpsych.ac.uk

Trust for the Study of Adolescence
No helpline, but its website gives information and useful links for parents and details of its published resources for parents.
23 New Road, Brighton BN1 1WZ
Telephone: 01273 693311 (ask for publications department)
www.tsa.uk.com/info

YoungMinds
This has a lot of useful links to other websites and is particularly aimed at young people.
102 Clerkenwell Road, London EC1M 5SA
Telephone: 020 7336 8445
Parents' information service: 0800 018 2138
www.youngminds.org.uk

Index